SEX

and the

PERFECT

LOVER

SEX

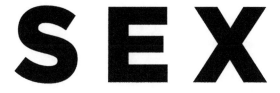

and the

PERFECT

LOVER

TAO, TANTRA, AND THE KAMA SUTRA

MABEL IAM

ATRIA BOOKS

New York London Toronto Sydney

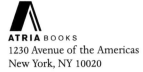

ATRIA B O O K S
1230 Avenue of the Americas
New York, NY 10020

Library of Congress Cataloging-in-Publication Data

Iam, Mabel.
   [Amante perfecto. English]
   Sex and the perfect lover : tao, tantra, and the Kama sutra / Mabel Iam.
     p. cm.
   Includes bibliographical references.
     1. Sex—Religious aspects—Taoism. 2. Sex—Religious aspects—Tantrism.
   3. Sex instruction—Religious aspects—Taoism. 4. Sex instruction—Religious
aspects—Tantrism. 5. Taoism. 6. Tantrism. I. Title.

   HQ61.I1613 2005
   306.7—dc22   2005053039

ISBN-13: 978-0-7432-8799-9
ISBN-10:   0-7432-8799-1

This Atria Books hardcover edition October 2005

10 9 8 7 6 5

ATRIA B O O K S is a trademark of Simon & Schuster, Inc.

Manufactured in the United States of America

For information about special discounts for bulk purchases,
please contact Simon & Schuster Special Sales:
1-800-456-6798 or business@simonandschuster.com.

Note: The ancient remedies portrayed in this book are historical references used for
educational purposes only. Recipes may not be used for profit. Contents are not in-
tended to diagnose, treat, prescribe, or replace recommendations made by health
professionals legally licensed and authorized to practice. New recipes must be applied in minimum doses to allow the body to assimilate them.

Any Internet references contained in this work are current at publication time, but
the publisher cannot guarantee that a specific location will continue to be main-
tained. Please refer to the publisher's website for links to authors' websites and other
sources.

7

Energy and Erotic Motion

As a form of yoga within the Hindu tradition, Tantra emphasizes the importance of knowing how vital energy circulates within the body in order to harmonize the circulation of this energy and develop its power.

The body is energy in action, but in order to develop the power of this vital energy, we have to know the points where this energy is concentrated and distributed.

According to Oriental teaching, when these points, referred to as *chakras*, become blocked—whether due to stress, emotional problems, inhibitions, phobias, or fear of contact, among other things—a person's sexual vitality diminishes considerably.

What Are Chakras?

They are seven centers distributed along the length of the body, connected to the glands that regulate the normal functioning of the respective areas of the body. When these centers malfunction, we are more susceptible to contracting various diseases that also affect our behavior and emotions.

Meditation and visualization help unblock these centers and harmonize their functions. The center corresponding to sexual energy is the one that is most often blocked.

How to Unblock the Sexuality Center

We can unblock our sexual energy by means of localization, relaxation, and motion. The more we relax and are aware of our emotional and sexual flow, the better we'll be able to control our personal power and enjoy our intimate relationships. Moving the areas of the body where sexual energy flows in a smooth and harmonious fashion helps us get to know that energy and enjoy it.

How to Enjoy the Erotic Rhythm

*The rhythm of pleasure became intertwined between
our legs to the rhythm of our hips.
The whole night we merged
in an erotic dance as though in a ritual.
The sweet friction of love's energy made us
shine in the darkness.
To our surprise, we discovered the sunrise
while we reflected our own light as if it were the moon.*

The purpose of these techniques is to respect, deepen, and stimulate the natural rhythms of the body. Through various motions in a state of relaxation, we can control and increase vitality and at the same time prevent muscle fatigue.

An Exercise to Prepare the Sexual Rhythm

This exercise can be performed individually or as a couple. It is performed standing up and walking.

First, you must completely relax your body. Focus your attention on your flow of energy while combining the rhythms of respiration with slow motions that use the weight of the body to move your arms and legs in an arch-like motion.

Then, with your legs apart and slightly bent, make short movements to observe each muscle's reflex and connection to respiration and circulation. Also note each muscle's direct relation to other parts of the body that relax or contract to enable the motion.

Usually, expansion motions are accompanied by an inhalation, and contraction motions by an exhalation. The flow of motions must be continuous.

The objective is to achieve "harmony of body and spirit" by being attentive to respiration and the way energy circulates throughout the body.

Dance and Joy: Sexual Rhythms, Step by Step

Men and women have different tempos of sexual response. If you wish for a maximum love connection with your partner, you need to experience the different rhythms, which range from wild, erotic rhythms to the softest and most tender cadences. Your sensations must become tuned to those of your lover, until both of you reach sexual fulfillment.

The First Rhythm Is the Sexual Impulse

This rhythm is directly related to the mutual attraction between the two partners. It is characterized by the seduction each partner provokes in the other.

The Second Rhythm Is Excitation

This tempo is spontaneous and is usually expressed more slowly in the woman and more quickly in the man. It depends exclusively on the erotic game that was induced by the first rhythm. It is important to personalize your ardor to stimulate your lover's erogenous zones.

The Third Rhythm Is the Orgasmic Rhythm

This rhythm is the result of the previous ones. Just like in a dance, lovers preserve an erotic energy of both instinctive and emotional encounters. This stage concentrates the mystery of the ecstasy of sexual rhythm.

The Fourth Rhythm Is Consummation

At this level an infinite explosion is achieved that transcends the limits of physical satisfaction and awakens the lovers' indescribable feelings. This burst, this explosive ecstasy, can only be attained through mutual surrender, while following the rhythm of love. When each lover adapts to the sexual response of the partner, the sexual act does not end with the orgasm—quite the contrary; after the temporary release, these techniques rekindle sexual pleasure.

The Game of Mirrors

Lovers can perform the Game of Mirrors exercise, which will help them appreciate the sensations of their partner. This technique is geared to polish your perceptions, so you can better appreciate your lover as a pleasurable object.

1. Lovers exchange sexual roles, by mutual agreement. This exercise is based on imitating the motions that are naturally performed by your partner in the course of the erotic game. First, one partner performs the active role and then the other will imitate him or her. This mirroring technique is the same technique used to learn any dancing move.

2. The marvelous thing about human beings while making love is that they can acquire knowledge and learn from different experiences by getting in contact with creativity and

pleasure. Astonishing results can be achieved by performing this exercise once a week and then once a month.

The couple that finds a unique rhythm transforms sexuality into the true art of loving.

8

Erotic Dance

Technique to Prepare for the Erotic Dance

Preparing for the erotic dance takes approximately an hour and consists of four steps. It is important to play music that is strong and vibrant, but is without lyrics, in order to avoid mental associations and memories. The purpose of this exercise is to induce mental silence.

First Step

For ten to fifteen minutes, relax and allow your body to move or quiver. Free yourself from all inhibitions. Feel how energy ascends from your feet throughout all of your body.

Relax your head and allow it to move wherever you wish. This can be done with your eyes open or closed.

Second Step

For ten to fifteen minutes, dance spontaneously as if you were a child. Let your body lead you inside that spontaneous rhythm.

Third Step

Close your eyes and be still, whether sitting down or standing up. The important thing is to be aware of anything you feel inside your body, such as restlessness, calm, tingling, or excitation.

Fourth Step

Quietly and with your eyes closed, notice the flow of your vital energy after moving. Breathe ever more slowly until you feel complete ecstasy with this natural dance of your body.

If the dance is performed as a couple, lovers ideally should try to coordinate their rhythms. They can touch each other and, with their legs apart, softly move their hips in mutual rhythm.

9

The Explosive Orgasm

We have already explored various elements that are conducive to achieving an intense sexual and spiritual relationship. All of these elements are steps that help us get in tune with both our own rhythms and with those of our partner. The steps also lead to achieving an explosive orgasm.

Before achieving an explosive orgasm, it is very pleasurable to softly massage your partner with a moisturizing lotion or cream on the lower back, the spine, and the inside surface of the arms and legs.

In men, the central area of their feet is particularly sensitive. The liver, which controls and releases the additional blood needed for erection, benefits directly from this stimulation.

How to Achieve the Explosion

In order to achieve a balance, the man must take in the woman's fluids. Taoist sexual discipline teaches men the "Great Liberation of the Three Peaks." This means that the man must absorb the secretions of the woman's lips and tongue, breasts, and vagina, or mons veneris. The man must lick up these secretions because, according to Taoists, they are very healthy. The man should use his tongue to stimulate the woman's mouth, breasts, the upper part of her pelvis, and the inside of her vagina.

How to Recognize the Signs that Indicate Sexual Enjoyment in Women

Practitioners of the Tao of Love assert that it is possible to recognize the degree of female pleasure by discovering the "Five Signs." If a lover pays attention to each of them, he will know how to make the right move at the right time.

1. When the woman's face blushes and her body temperature rises, her partner should start to play tenderly.

2. The man should penetrate the woman when he observes that her nipples are hard and small drops of sweat appear around her nose.

3. If he notices dryness in her throat and lips, he should thrust more vigorously.

4. When female lubrication turns slippery, the man should achieve the deep explosion. He needs to keep moving his pelvis while penetration lasts and not stop. He should softly squeeze the woman's body against his, but each time with more insistence.

5. The last sign will be the secretion of a viscous fluid on the woman's thighs. This indicates that she has reached the high tide of orgasmic explosion. At this moment, the man should begin breathing exercises in order to withhold ejaculation for a longer time, which makes it possible to employ different positions in search of the supreme pleasure.

10

The Body and Its Colors

The Tao of Sex and Its Colors

If you fill your life with the proper colors, you will be able to change your feelings and your perceptions and noticeably improve each sexual experience.

Sex and Colors

Sexual rituals have long been performed by using various supporting elements—from candles of different colors to special garments whose colors, textures, and styles varied depending on the ritual's origin.

Nothing escapes the power of the colors in a rainbow. In our daily lives, we usually spend considerable time choosing the colors we use to paint each room of our house, and we recognize the energy emitted by the colors of crystals and stones that shine in earrings or other jewels.

The discipline of chromotherapy studies the effects of colors on people. By using some of these findings, it is possible to reestablish the natural power of our energy centers by visualizing specific colors, or by using illumination, choosing colors that strengthen and reinforce our erogenous zones.

"Nothing is true or false—it all depends on the color of the glass you look through," says a Spanish proverb, and it contains more than a grain of truth. Colors are nothing but light beams reflected or emitted by the objects we see. This luminous radiation has the power to exert a healing influence through the various energy channels in our body.

Likewise, working internally and externally with colors modifies our disposition and the "waves" we emit.

The Purpose of Visualizing Each Color

Yellow

Yellow is a natural stimulant of emotions. It helps harmonize wishes and desires and make them come true.

Blue

Blue is a cold color that relieves anxiety and helps control attacks of obsessive sexual attraction.

White

White is used in purification rituals and is related to the cleanliness that should precede a sexual relation or a love union.

Navy Blue

Blue is a great spiritual generator. It magnetizes people's environments, thereby attracting states of peace, protection, and safety.

Gray

The neutral color par excellence, gray is useful for creating environments that foster an objective understanding of what's happening around us.

Brown

Brown is associated with the persistence and patience of those who help us grow spiritually.

Orange

Orange has a soothing effect that acts directly on the central nervous system and increases our attention span.

Black

Black absorbs light. It is associated with female energy and with the dark side of the Tao symbol, but its effect may vary depending on how it is used.

Red

Red symbolizes sexual power. It increases eroticism and provides strength and endurance. It fills the blood with oxygen and clears its toxins.

Pink

Pink preserves love in sexual relationships and fuses love and erotic passion into a bond.

Green

Green is associated with nature and living energy. Its hypnotic vibrations bring calm to the body and mind.

Violet

Violet is the manifestation of the spirit, which is why it is the color used to transform negative emotions and thoughts.

Multicolor Pleasure

When you think of two lovers, you never imagine them vibrating together in black and white. What color excites you?

Colors produce an energy vibration that acts on different planes, but the art of making love requires more than a mere game with colors. The culmination of pleasure is marked by a variety of colors felt only by those who are willing to experiment with the various hues.

Colors and Sexual Motivation

Colors express moods and emotions that are directly related to concrete psychic meanings. They also clearly exert a physiological effect. Whenever we have problems with our partner due to a lack of sexual desire or because there isn't a strong erotic chemistry, we can use different colors to increase pleasure to its utmost level.

The most common practice is to use colors as part of the environment's decor. For example, to foster moments of pleasure, you can place a specially colored light in the room. Red symbolizes passion, vitality, and strength. Orange is a source of refreshing energy and is useful in solving communication problems. It also enhances the physical connection. The use of various hues of red and other bright colors in lingerie accentuates the female form.

Visible Impact

We must be particularly aware of how we prepare ourselves for the ritual of passion—what clothes, makeup, or other enhancements we choose to wear before making love. Certain color combinations continue to exert a subliminal effect on our lover's mind after the moment of intimacy.

These colors cause the same magnetism as the colors that are used to control city traffic. They are colors that should stand out from our surroundings to increase our lover's focus on our body and the situation at hand. Here are some possible combinations:

Black and yellow
Green and white
Red and white
Blue and white

Incorporating any of these color combinations into the environment where the moment of intimacy is to take place will increase and enhance the visual impact. Start with the bed sheets and include any bodily accessories. When a couple is having problems, the first impact a change in the environment can have is to arouse interest, curiosity, and finally excitation.

The Inner Circle and Its Colors

A human being is a bundle of energies as vibrant as colors. If we have a positive relationship with our partner, an effective technique is to concentrate on a protective energy before beginning foreplay. Already in the nude, both partners can visualize each other wrapped in a spiral of a particular color, depending on the effect they wish to achieve.

The Dragonfly

To perform the sexual act in this position, the partners must lie on their sides on a flexible and comfortable place, such as a bed or a sofa. The woman lies on her side with her back turned to her partner, and he mounts her from the back. This way, the bodies fit each other in a position that is ideal for very affectionate couples who enjoy demonstrating the tenderness they feel toward each other.

With a bit of skill combined with much excitement, the woman takes her flexed outer leg and places it on the man's coccyx, thus opening the door to pleasure. The man penetrates her by using his lover's leg as an erotic lever bracing on the support of his hip.

The flattering words the man is able to whisper in his partner's ear, because it is so close to his mouth, provide the perfect compliment to achieve the utmost delight, in addition to ardent kisses. The woman, upon just listening to him, lets herself be taken over by the rhythm of his kisses, while she shows her lover all the effects his potency has on her through her expressions of intense pleasure.

Penetration goes halfway, which is why the pleasure is enhanced by the desire to make penetration deep and cause the explosion of the most exciting orgasm.

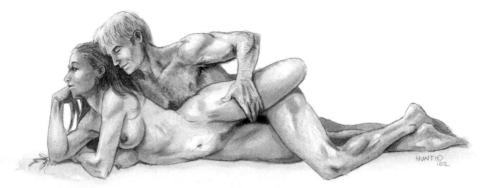

The Screw

Nothing is more advisable to a woman who finds it difficult to reach orgasm than assuming positions that press on the clitoris while the vagina is penetrated. Orgasm always comes in this position, and multiple experiences of pleasure become concrete and unforgettable feelings for the woman.

She lies down by the edge of the bed and places her flexed legs to one side of her body (each woman will know which side is most comfortable for her). This enables her to keep the clitoris trapped between the best allies she has to reach the prized orgasm—the labia of her vagina.

The woman can contract and relax that entire region, while the man, kneeling in front of her, penetrates her softly. To turn this position into a true delicacy, it is suitable for the man, while penetrating her, to caress her breasts and for the woman to groan with pleasure to arouse her partner.

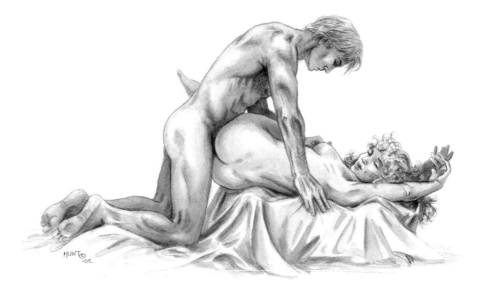

The Amazon

This position puts the woman in a totally active position. She places herself on top of the man and sets the rhythm of the sexual relation by bracing her feet on the floor. It is ideal for active women who are a bit domineering and like to set the sexual rhythm in a relationship.

For the man, this is an extraordinary experience because in this position he can incorporate the yin energy, which is more passive, and in addition be able to relax in the course of the sexual act. In turn he can touch her breasts and pull the hair of his mate while she moves.

The visual angle made possible by this variation is one of the most exciting angles for the man, since he is able to see close at hand each thrust he performs on his partner. And the woman will get much pleasure from the idea of knowing that she is in control of the sexual act and that the man knows it.

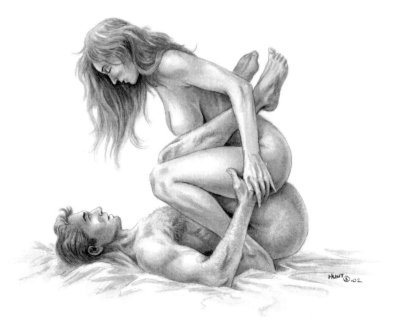

The Easy Chair

Leaning on a big, comfortable cushion or pillow, the man sits with his legs flexed and a bit open. The woman sits comfortably on the space he's formed with his body. In this position, the protective feelings of both partners come to the fore.

Assisted by his arms and hands, the man finds the satisfactory point of encounter for both and places his partner on his erection, controlling the sexual rhythm.

Her legs are braced on the shoulders of her mate, who has his head trapped and wrapped between her thighs. The man can touch her clitoris while he forcefully grabs her by her waist.

The distance between the faces and the daring aspect of this proposal endow this position with an extremely sensual quality.

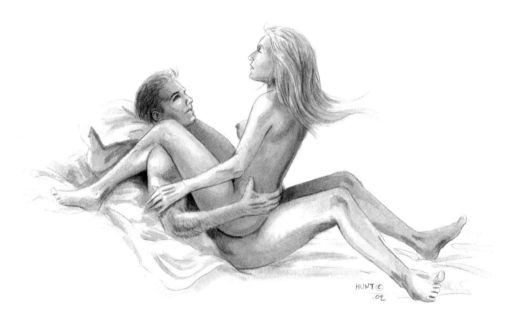

The Sleepy Woman

The woman lies on her side and the man mounts her from the back in order to penetrate her. She stretches a leg backward and wraps it around his waist. This position is ideal for well-endowed men who always had experiences in the traditional position, and for very flexible women who want to place their whole body at the disposal of their mate.

Additionally, it fulfills several longings of fantasy-driven minds. First of all, she is in front of him and at the same time has access to his face and neck, and he has access to her face and neck. Secondly, he has comfortable access to her clitoris and is able to touch and feel the breasts of his lover.

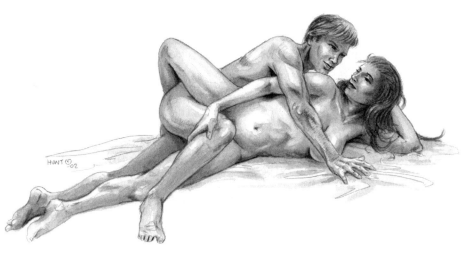

The Surprise

In this position the man must be standing up to grab the woman from behind, penetrate her, and at the same time take her by the hips in a sensual manner and with a certain degree of domination. She relaxes her whole body and places her hands on the floor in an attitude of surrender and of confidence in her partner. The man "surprises" the woman from behind, setting the erotic rhythm almost completely.

For her, pleasure is concentrated because of the opening angle of the vagina, which, being narrow, provokes a very intense, pleasant sensation. For him, the most powerful sensation expands upward from the glans, which comes into and out of the vagina at will and caresses the clitoris in the most daring moves as it comes out. In addition, the man's visual field covers her anus, her buttocks, and her back, zones that are very erogenous for many people. The domination exerted by the man on the woman together with her complete relaxation may foster playfulness in the man, who while seducing his lover is able to play around with her anus. If she already knows the experience, the woman may approach the sensation of pleasure caused by her lover's anal penetration.

This position is ideal for those who love the most savage and primitive forms of sexual intercourse.

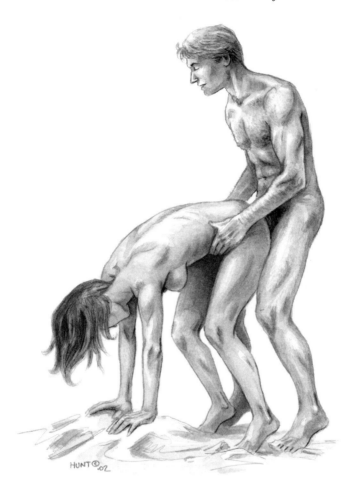

The Medusa

The partners should kneel on a comfortable surface, though not as soft as a bed. In this position, the man surrenders to the woman's will. She descends on his penis and introduces it into her vagina whenever she wishes. Before penetration, they may kiss, rub each other's breasts, hug, caress each other's back, and place the glans in her vagina and rub it against the clitoris, creating a pleasant and very different sensation, an almost unique one. After being very much desired, the penetration will come with infinite pleasure at the end.

In the course of the love act, if he can't surrender patiently to her moves, he'll be able to set the rhythm by grabbing her by the waist and drawing her body to his.

Since the partners are face to face, this offers the exciting opportunity to observe each other, rejoice together, talk, and kiss each other on the mouth until achieving the much desired orgasm.

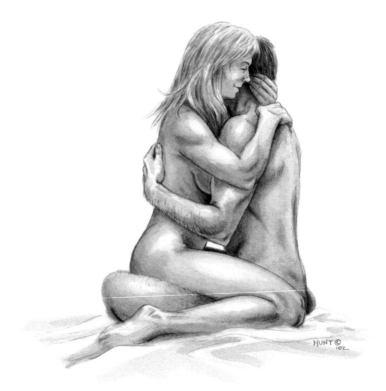

The Fusion

In this position, the man sits down, tilting his body slightly backward, supporting it by bracing his hands on the bed on each side of his body. The legs may be stretched or bent, depending on the partners' comfort. The heads of both partners should be relaxed. The woman assumes the active role on this occasion, passing her legs over her lover and supporting herself by bracing her arms behind her body.

To be totally successful in this position, stimulation must be intense, since during penetration this position prevents manual contact and contact of the mouths of the partners.

The woman sets the rhythm and establishes the genital encounter with a very marked motion. It is essential to have the clitoris take full advantage of the impacts with her lover's body in order to maintain the excitement until the moment she decides to explode with pleasure, provided her lover keeps the rhythm with a good erection.

The look is a fundamental component, but so is sensual and provocative communication, since erotic words provide a very strong sexual charge to the love act. Both resources (looks and words) can be unbelievable weapons used to enjoy this position and achieve a complete "fusion."

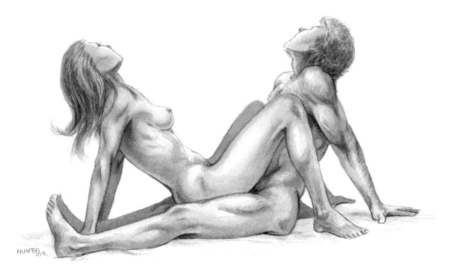

Possession

As its name indicates, this position is captivating and has a certain degree of suggestion, especially for the woman. The man can use all his sexual magnetism and enjoy his own energy in this posture.

The woman lies on her back with her legs open, waiting for her partner to penetrate her, while he sits down and holds her by her shoulders to regulate the motion. Their legs become intertwined in a sensual and pleasant manner.

The male organ penetrates and withdraws, deviating its movement downward, since the body of the woman is slightly higher than the body of the man. He can then explore the woman's G-Spot and all of her genital area in order to give his partner everything she loves.

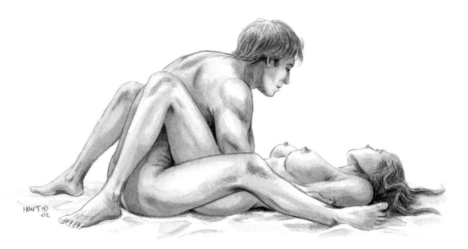

Face to Face

This is the most classic and universal position known in the art of making love. It provides a lot of security for couples in which the woman needs the man's bodily, sexual, and emotional protection.

The state of being face to face makes for a large number of variations to this position, which makes it an attractive and exciting one. The mobility of the hands, the closeness of the faces, and the comfort of the bodies are some of the advantages that made it famous.

The lovers should not fear trying new types of contact during the love act in this position. She can touch her mate's glutei and anal areas. He can rub her clitoris or allow her to do it herself. The legs of both partners may be closer together in order to create a certain degree of difficulty in the penetration.

This is a position that many lovers identify with the love and romance they experienced at the beginning of their life as a couple. It is worth it to experience it at the various stages of their sexual life and to profit to the utmost from all its advantages.

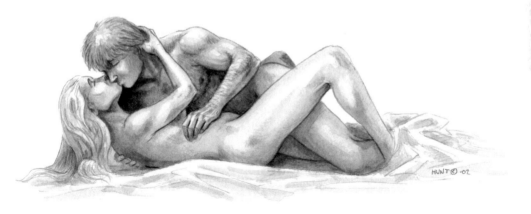

Face-to-Face Variation

This is the same classic position, but the difference, perhaps more exciting, is that the woman assumes the active and dominating role. This variation of the "face to face" is a position that favors women who can't reach orgasm easily because they need a very active and direct stimulation of the clitoris and labia.

In this variation of the love act, the woman can rub her clitoris against the body of her lover, and, due to her dominating position, can move easily and with greater bodily freedom. Additionally, the man can touch with joy his mate's buttocks and play around with his fingers in search of the complete satisfaction of both partners.

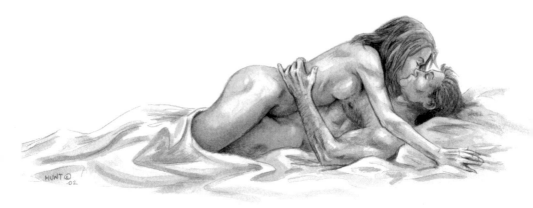

The three basic types of manipulation are soft rubbing, kneading, and friction.

Soft Rubbing

Oil is applied in this type of rubbing to help you get to know your lover's body. You place your hands flat on your mate's back with your fingers relaxed and softly slide them down, trying to locate potential tension nodes. Pressure should usually be increased as your hands near the area of the heart. This has a relaxing effect, which is felt at the nerves located under the skin.

Kneading

Kneading consists of energetic motions that imitate the kneading of dough, and is particularly helpful for releasing accumulated tension. This type of manipulation is indicated for the more muscular regions. To do it well, you must press the skin between your thumb and your fingers and sink the thumb into the muscle mass. With your fingers, push the muscle toward you again. Move your hands, alternating between one and the other, pressing, pushing, and lifting the skin.

Friction

Friction consists of pressing rather small, specific areas, which induces a very pleasant, restful sensation. It is important to push the tip of the thumb downward and perform short rotational motions to achieve a deeper penetration. Friction has an analgesic effect and stimulates blood flow.

29

Sexual Magic

Introduction to Sexual Magic

Sexual magic leads to the union of body and soul. It transcends sex, space, and time. Sexual magic allows us to eliminate the negative aspects of a love relationship. It brings about a full enjoyment of life and a state of ecstasy that expands beyond the limits of our bodies until it achieves harmony with the universe.

When we speak of sexual magic, the reader usually associates it with casting "love spells" or, in the worst cases, using exotic recipes and secretly placing them in the food of some victim we want to win over. Some people may compare sexual magic with the degree of hypnosis or suggestion exerted by Count Dracula on the innocent Lucy.

In reality, sexual magic is the metaphysical explanation of how energy forces interact in a sexual relationship. They are the energies that attract and repel each other in the game of love.

When we talk about male or female energies as necessary elements for every sexual act, it is important to understand that female energy does not belong exclusively to women, nor does male energy belong exclusively to men. Both are part of our system. We all have them regardless of our gender.

Why does attraction take place between two bodies? The exchange of hormones is not the only thing that produces a pleasurable sexual contact. In a sexual act, both feelings and mental energy exert their influence. According to the magic ritual, a state of meditation before sex clears away the emotions that might have blocked the relationship. The mind becomes a sexual organ and contributes to the optimum workings of sexual magic.

The magical techniques used to get rid of negative thoughts and emotions are performed before and during intercourse. Sexual magic is not an action we mechanically perform, but rather a conscious exploration of our sexual and spiritual potential.

In order to implement these techniques, we must learn to eliminate fear. Ignorance of the limits of our sexual potential can provoke negative fantasies in a person or in the bond that binds a couple. We need to develop the feminine and masculine aspects of our inner selves. Each person, individually or with a partner, can attain an ever higher degree of ecstasy, which can reach an explosive state.

How to Practice Sexual Magic

If you do the exercise as a couple, it will be unforgettable for both of you. The lovers should sit down in front of each other and look at each other with the same trust and intimacy they experience when they look in a mirror, with the same attitude as when they see their own face in the morning.

Observe the other person without prejudice, as if that other person were a part of you and different only in appearance. If you are both undressed in a quiet place, the experience is much more powerful. If you start to feel the need to touch each other, that is because you are still avoiding the deep look I'm proposing. Observation must be, each time, ever more innocent. Try to get rid of sexual bodily perceptions and any emotions that may arise. Try to feel that way until you feel the other person as being a part of yourself.

If you do this by yourself, sit down in front of the mirror and perform the exercise the same way. It's possible that looking at your own body may also produce excitation. That's okay, because it shows that your vital energy is acting in a natural way. Don't repress your feelings—just observe without making any movement.

When you both feel that your minds are empty of the compulsion to act, then you can start to approach each other. At that moment, close your eyes.

Now listen to your hearts with your eyes closed. Without taking your own pulse, each of you should try to listen to the beating of your own heart, breathing and relaxing each time you release air. Become aware of the state of your body and try to perceive your partner's body intuitively without opening your eyes. This task is called *centering* and is an exercise that precedes magical meditation.

The centering state is essential, and it is also very easy to achieve. The objective is to train the body to be able to focus the mind wherever the will chooses. To do this, you both must learn to be present and relaxed and to get rid of the emotions that block sexual performance.

If you don't achieve centering after twenty minutes, you can still attain an optimum state by repeating the following affirmation mentally: "My relaxation is complete for the enjoyment of the spirit."

Magical Meditation: The Path to Sexual Ecstasy

"A man and a woman . . .
The man is the eagle that flies.
The woman is the nightingale that sings.
To fly is to master space.

To sing is to conquer the soul.
The man is a temple.
The woman is the altar.
Before the temple we uncover ourselves;
before the altar we kneel down . . .
The man is where the Earth ends.
The woman is where Heaven starts."

—*Victor Hugo*

Relaxation exercises are part of the sexual magic technique. The first step is to concentrate before meditating, either individually or as a couple, to achieve mental and emotional control before having sex.

Prior to learning the next steps of this technique, we have to ask ourselves: How can we manage to concentrate on something so perfect as divinity if at the same time our whole body is excited and we feel the need to touch our partner?

The answer is not easy because, for thousands of years, men and women dutifully denied their sexuality and underestimated the energy of the sex act. But it is not that complicated either—you just need to feel a deep love for your partner and a great need to explore your sexual power beyond the limits of your imagination.

The act of learning to meditate ought to hold the same attraction for us as, for example, making love for the first time. It is an endearing, spiritual, and loving adventure, but the most important thing is to know that once one has been initiated in this technique, it is impossible to go back to the original state.

Now find a private place where you continue to follow all of the previous steps. Once you achieve this relaxed state, you should then center on your breathing. With each inhalation you must count to three, withhold the air, and exhale slowly. Your breathing must be almost imperceptible.

Once you achieve this state, locate in the area of your heart the most perfect and ideal image of what you wish to attain with your partner. If you can't visualize it, recreate internally a feeling or sensation that you would like to experience, without any prejudices. You should not see the image outside of you, as if it were projected onto a screen, but rather very vividly and with the full sensation of immediate experience.

After completing this concentration and creative visualization, you can take a few minutes to comment on the experience with your partner, without making comparisons.

If you performed the exercise individually, you can write about each visualization, as well as how the clarity, power, and strength of your meditation is evolving.

The success of this meditation can be observed when you experience greater control, confidence, and, above all, a feeling of happiness, in all aspects of your life.

The Keys to Opening and Developing Sexual Magic

To magically create our own universe, we need magical elements, such as light, space, time, and the channel for divine action—the human being. But the most important thing is not to forget that all human beings are equal or similar to our divine creator. This is the basis for the magic. Here are the keys to sexual magic.

Space

With your partner, look within your home for a place that is reasonably quiet. It does not have to be your bedroom. Any place where you know no one is going to bother you will do. Once there, get rid of all possible interferences, from the telephone to the television. Try to ventilate the environment and spread a soft aroma by burning myrrh or sandalwood incense. Turn off the lights. If possible, lightly illuminate the environment with a red candle.

Centering Yourself

Once you have succeeded in becoming centered, both of you should undress, which is also the best thing to do to get rid of your bodily inhibitions.

Perform the Protection Ritual

The first magical exercise you can try is a simple protection ritual. All you have to do is visualize a circle of light around your head that gradually descends throughout your body. The color of the energy with which you should meditate is brilliant white. Then imagine that same circle around yourself and around your partner's body. If you are by yourself, you can imagine it the same way, but you must feel as if your partner were present, sitting in front of you. Then you can expand the circle and surround the whole place, and then the whole house, until it finally surrounds the whole planet with its brilliant white light.

Focusing and Deepening

Try to focus mentally on the idea that this circle is protecting you and that nothing can happen to you, that the world is in harmony and complete fulfillment. Try to feel the ecstasy inside you, the peace and security of a world illuminated by a white light. If you still experience difficulties visualizing, try to think as if you were "daydreaming," but under your conscious control. It's like being reasonably attentive to what goes on around you, and still continuing to dream of your lover or partner or the whole universe surrounded by beauty and love.

With time and practice, you will be able to visualize anything you desire. You'll be able to practice a meditation that is more easily controlled each time, but it is not necessary for you to achieve this at the beginning. Try to maintain the state of ecstasy, control your breathing, and assess your state of relaxation on a permanent basis.

Erogenous Points

Now that you feel more relaxed, try to center on your heart, imagining that your mate is lying down. Visualize your partner and yourself as if you both were the God or Goddess of Love, and with this incomparable sensation imagine yourself caressing your lover's body. Think intuitively about the places where this person can feel the most pleasure. Don't get ahead of yourself—only caress your partner in your imagination. Don't focus on the parts of your lover's body that you like, but rather on those that you know are most pleasurable to your partner.

Intensification

With your eyes still closed, ask yourself: What is the level of intensity that I need in order to excite my lover? How far do I have to go in my exploration? What force or pressure do I have to exert?

> Try to feel the ecstasy of the other person, and vibrate inside your mate's body as if it were your own.
>
> Don't lose your concentration.
>
> Don't open your eyes.
>
> Don't lose your level of relaxation.

Continue performing this meditation until ecstasy becomes completely explosive.

30

Relationships with Love

The Seven Golden Rules

Our thoughts are creative—they create everything around us, especially everything that we focus on and comprehend. Sometimes our thoughts do this consciously and sometimes, in most cases, unconsciously. So if we want to change the world around us and our relationships, we have to start with our thoughts:

1. Our thoughts have the power to transform.
2. You are and have what you think and believe.
3. We have many thoughts per second; we need to make them conscious.
4. We can change everything we think.
5. We must be attentive to what we wish for and think . . .
6. . . . to master our thoughts and not allow them to control us.
7. We have to exercise our thoughts daily—we need time and space to focus our energy to transform, to learn, and to evolve.

Creative Visualization Techniques

If we observe and investigate our internal world, we'll discover to what point our thinking is creative and powerful. To attain this excellent creative visualization, there are two steps that must be followed:

First Step: Complete Breathing

Complete breathing consists of working with the lungs and the abdomen to achieve a proper deep respiration. You must be lying down on the floor in a comfortable place where you won't be interrupted for about fifteen to thirty minutes.

At the beginning, until your breathing is natural and fluid, it is advisable to perform this exercise with your body at rest.

Pay attention to your thoughts and let them pass on as if they were a shower of energy—don't identify with any of them. After a few minutes of relaxation, place one hand on your abdomen and the other one on your chest. Let out all the air softly through your nose, emptying your lungs completely. Try to keep your lungs empty for a few seconds. Inhale slowly, inflating only your abdomen until you fill up the lower part of your lungs—without exerting yourself, you'll feel how your diaphragm expands downward. At this moment, the lower and middle parts of your lungs are full of air.

Before exhaling, take advantage of this moment and empty your mind of all your thoughts and imagine that you're also getting rid of all your daily tensions and emotions. Then move the air to the upper area of your lungs and, little by little, let it out.

Repeat this process for a minimum of ten minutes.

Second Step: Mental Concentration and Creative Visualization

Before starting the visualization exercise, have everything written down in detail so you have a clear view of what you want to achieve. You should clearly define each affirmation that you want to come true. For example:

1. Improve communication with your partner during dinner.

2. Understand your children better during the month of June.

3. Not have any problems at work today.

Let's consider the first example:

Visualize your partner and you sitting at home for dinner. When you do the exercise, don't imagine that you're watching a movie in your mind—try to feel, with all your senses, what you're visualizing as if you were really doing it.

Then imagine a scene in which there is little communication between the two of you, and scratch out that mental image with a huge X. Add to this imaginary action the word *canceled*.

Then imagine you both having a friendly and affectionate dinner, with all the details you want included. Ideally you should do two creative visualizations a day until they come true. Once a visualization has become real, keep working on new ones, but never visualize more than two images a day.

The mind is very literal and orderly. Always remember that if we have the capacity to dream, it is because we also have the ability to make those dreams come true.

Relationships with Love

Creating relationships with love is to participate in the celebration of love that the universe offers each day. We have inside ourselves a dark corner that keeps us from enjoying life. We can illuminate this corner with mental clarity and a willing heart. Life is a beautiful invitation. Do you want to enjoy all aspects of love? Don't procrastinate. It all depends on you.

The Path Toward a Mind of Light

Visualization enables you to have a harmonious relationship with your own self and with others. It consists of four steps:

Clearing the Mind

The purpose of clearing the mind is to quiet the roaring stream of thoughts that flows all the time. This objective is achieved through good, full breathing.

Observing the Mind

For visualization to be effective, you must be attentive to the thoughts that crop up in your mind. When you lose your concentration, relax again and pay attention to your breathing. A very interesting meditation involves realizing how the chain of thoughts operates, how thoughts are linked to each other.

Disciplining the Mind

In this step we have to penetrate the contents of thought, and see how one thought leads to another and then on to another and how they are all linked. You don't have to get involved with these thoughts; just observe how the process takes place without paying too much attention to what the actual subject of thought is, because oftentimes it is emotional energy that finds its way to the mental plane.

Affirmations

Discipline enables the mind to use affirmations. Affirmations are one of the most powerful tools at the mind's disposal, and are achieved by fixing the affirmation and visualizing it clearly. An affirmation can also be repeated like a mantra. Ideally, each affirmation should be repeated fifteen minutes a day until it comes true.

The Different Kinds of Relationships and Emotional Energy

The world is full of positive and negative energy. Emotions are one aspect of it. There is a separation between emotions that are incorrectly called negative and emotions that are incorrectly called positive. Emotions are simply energies in motion. What makes them positive or negative is what we do with them and the effects they have on our relationships. Anger, hate, and fear are emotions that are called negative because they block us, make us ill, and torment us. Love, hope, and affection are called positive because they heal us, give us relief, and protect us. All emotions are part of life, but how can we manage our emotions?

Learning to Have Relationships with Love

To be able to love, we have to control our fears and the negative energy they produce. The following steps help create a good internal basis:

1. The mind cannot entertain two thoughts at the same time; therefore, when the first negative thought comes up, clear your mind and cancel that thought. You will discipline your mind and learn to focus on the positive.

2. Try to discover the source of each negative emotion that crops up. This will lead you to self-knowledge and wisdom.

3. Avoid judging or censuring others. It is better to try to reinforce and strengthen the positive we see in others; otherwise, the finger you point at them tomorrow may be pointed back at you. If you strive to see the good both in you and others, very soon you'll be much happier.

4. Living in darkness is not the same as remaining in a dark chamber—it means not being able to see the reality of life in harmony and light. You may choose to live always

in darkness, but if you tire of it, you can turn on the light. Seeing clearly is a mental exercise that is achieved by gaining an awareness of all your positive emotions until you discover the best in you.

5. Observe role models or attitudes that you would like to imitate. Having a positive role model can be of help, provided you don't idealize that person.

6. Choose which emotions you want for your relationships. You should have control over your life and your emotions. Try to observe each stimulus that comes to you, how you react, and what effect it produces in you. This mechanism will provide you with permanent self-awareness.

7. Bring to mind all opportunities open to you. When you believe you're hurt by the effect of your negative emotions, make a list of all the positive ways in which you could respond to this situation. This system creates a protective mechanism that will never fail you.

8. Visualize this list and work on the daily affirmations until you achieve your goal.

Remember how many times you have lost your footing while you were on the path of insecurity and fear. Now is the time to tread along the path of love. Your perfect guide will be the sweet whisperings that always spring from your heart.